**Understanding Food: Nutritiona
Healthy, Diet-Fre**

By Jicotea Kinsella

Text Copyright © 2015 Jicotea Kinsella

All Rights Reserved

Table of Contents

Contents

Introduction

Chapter 1- Importance of a Healthy Diet

Chapter 2- Suggested Nutritional Requirements from the Food Groups

Chapter 3- Serving Sizes

Chapter 4- Understanding Proteins and Amino Acids

Chapter 5- Healthy Eating Guidelines

Chapter 6- Summary

Introduction

We understand that life can be fast paced, hectic and chaotic at times, making it difficult for you to plan out your meals such that you make sensible food choices. However, when you have the right information on the nutritional facts of your favorite meals, and you know what it does to your health and well-being, we are sure you'll agree that a little planning goes a long way in building a healthy and fit body. In fact, nutrition plays a decisive role in shaping your personality and physique. A healthy diet that aims at good nutrition can determine how healthy you are and fit you stay. In addition to this, it lowers your risk of chronic ailments and assists a healthy environment for pregnant mothers and their babies. What's more, healthy eating habits ensure you perform at your best, every single day of your life. This guide addresses the nutritional facts of your favorite foods while highlighting the benefits of a healthy and nutritious diet.

It has been observed that most food guides focus on drawing attention and addressing information in two ways. Graphical representations of the food pyramid and nutrition table help to highlight key information on statistics and numbers. The images are quick to assimilate and memorize and are designed to help you remember long and complex information. The other method that works in coordination with the previous one adopts an advisory model and guides you through ways and means to improve eating habits and general health. In this document, we have predominantly used words and information to help drive down the importance of nutrition and its impacts on your body and good health.

Rather than memorizing the food pyramid's general recommendations, we feel better off with an arsenal of specific information about health and food. Making healthy choices goes far beyond servings from the food groups.

We all have individual and unique food choices that are influenced by our taste, appetite, environment, and bodily requirements. In addition to this, our childhood practices, family culture and social interactions also influence our choice of food and nutrition. Ignoring these influences is counter-productive when working towards healthier eating habits. Rather, we should embrace our appetite and cultural backgrounds when it comes to food.

At a time when an average youngster suffers risks from diseases such as diabetes, hypertension, and high cholesterol, understanding your family's health history and your own biological disposition towards certain ailments can help you make sensible food choices. Once you make it a habit to eat right and healthy, you'll notice a great deal of energy and good health.

Chapter 1- Importance of a Healthy Diet

The importance of a healthy diet that provides adequate nutrition cannot be emphasized enough. Providing healthy diets to children helps them grow physically strong and mentally sharp. Ensuring they have a well-balanced and nutritious diet helps promote superior performance in school. Adults also benefit from a healthy and nutritious lifestyle; they stay healthy and lead a more fulfilled and complete life. This in turn increases their productivity, enabling them to lead a happy, long life.

Healthy food choices help you stay in control of your body, reducing the risk of many diseases and ailments. What's more, it can help you stay fit, making you feel and look younger. Well, we reckon that is a good enough reason to start paying attention to your diet!

Food and the nutrients contained in food give you the energy you require to perform daily activities. Having a diet that is well-balanced in nutrition and goodness will give you the stamina to run a long and successful race. On the contrary, fad and crash diets can wreak havoc on your good health and well-being. They snatch you off your physiological balance and leave you feeling tired, lethargic and completely depleted of energy. Today, when about 70 % of the world's population is either on the verge of starting or ending a fad diet plan, it becomes all the more imperative for us to address the importance of consuming food that is adequately nutritious. Our choices and decisions influence the world around us. It is the responsibility of every adult to make lifestyle and food choices that are both beneficial to them as well as their children.

So, we've spoken about the importance of nutrition and a bit about the benefits we stand to gain from it. We understand that the food we consume is converted into nutrients by our body. It is then used to supply us with energy to carry on daily activities. While our body is equipped to convert foods into nutrients and hence make most of the nutrients required on its own, there are a few essential nutrients that our body cannot make on its own. These nutrients are essential for our body's to function and hence, must be consumed through the food we eat. These essential nutrients include vitamins, minerals, amino acids of certain types and healthy fatty acids. In addition, it's important that we also consume a certain amount of carbohydrates in our daily meals and include adequate fiber. Each of these essential nutrients has a specific role to play in our well-being. They all collectively contribute to the overall health and primary functions of our bodies.

While most of us have partial information on certain nutrients, we sometimes fail to understand and recognize the larger picture of it all. For example, we've been told right from when we were young that consuming calcium works great for building strong and sturdy bones. However, many of us fail to recognize that there are several other nutrients that along with calcium work at developing and maintaining a healthy bone structure. In this book, we've tried to shed some light onto the other, lesser-known beneficial nutrients.

Food is measured in calories which are an indicator of the amount of energy it supplies when burned in the body. On an average, carbohydrates and protein contain four calories for every gram. Fats amount to a little more than twice the calories of carbohydrates with nine calories for every gram of fat. Alcohol is also high in energy and amounts to seven calories for every gram (few sips) consumed. Obviously, consuming food that is high in fat infers that you are consuming a high-calorie meal. A high-calorie meal requires higher levels of physical activity to burn off the additional energy consumed.

Your food consumption should be proportionate to your energy requirements. In general, children have a highly physically active life and require more energy to lead their lives and develop into healthy adults. They also burn calories and energy more quickly than adults, so they require a diet that is both nutritious and higher in calories. Adults, with the exception of individuals involved in sports or regular strenuous physical activity, require fewer calories to carry out their daily tasks. The more calories you consume, the more energy you end up accumulating. If the energy is adequately spent through physical activity, you end up being appropriately built in weight. However, if the calories consumed exceed the energy spent, you end up gaining weight, which can lead to several health problems in the long run. In addition to this, it is not enough to just consume the required number of calories in a day. It's important you consume the right kind of calories from the right kind of food sources for a healthy and balanced lifestyle. It is no wonder then that people who wish to lose weight are often advised to cut back calories while increasing their physical activities. The goal with any weight loss plan should include improving overall health, so it is important to look a little further than simple calorie counting. Having a well-balanced and nutritious diet can help you overcome any weight issues you might be suffering with, while helping you to reach your ideal weight and health.

The next few chapters highlight the importance of nutrition and its role in preventing health deficiencies. While a majority of people might be well informed about the adverse effects of malnutrition, fewer know that consuming nutrients in excess can also lead to health problems. For this reason, we suggest you pay attention to the quantity and type of nutrients suggested in this book. Doing so will help you lead a healthier and potentially disease-free life.

Chapter 2- Suggested Nutritional Requirements from the Food Groups

The recommended dietary allowances (RDAs) by the Food and Nutrition Board provide nutritional allowances that when followed, help maintain a healthy and nutritious lifestyle. The dietary allowance clearly outlines the recommended levels of nutrition to be consumed across all ages and both genders. This information provides a useful overview of what the average person requires, but it is important to remember that these suggestions do not work for everyone. A more personalized approach to nutrition will yield better results. However, the RDAs are based on sound research and will provide you with a great starting point in your quest for a healthier life.

Start by Reading Food Labels

People who are even slightly food and weight conscious will look out for the food labels printed on the back of most food items. This label is designed to provide information on the nutritional facts of a particular food; helping you select foods that meet the recommended dietary allowances. While most foods come with printed nutritional labels, there are a few exceptions. Beverages such as coffee and tea do not contain any specific nutritional value and might not come with the nutritional label printed on it. Foods available at restaurants, or foods that are made fresh to order might not come with a nutritional label unless it's printed on the menu itself. While the rule to provide nutritional labels is specific to processed food in particular, other food groceries such as raw food, fruits, vegetables, meats, and freshly cooked food might or might not come with the food label depending on the manufacturer's decision to do so or not. While food labels can provide a snapshot of the nutritional value of foods, they do not offer a complete picture. For this reason, the nutrition facts on food labels should serve as a general guide when selecting food products. In addition to the nutrition facts, get in the habit of reading the ingredient lists, too. This will help you become more aware of what you are eating and is a huge step in the right direction when it comes to your health.

The Five Food Groups

According to the United States Department of Agriculture (USDA), food can be categorized into five specific food groups. Consuming a variety of foods from each food group acts as the building blocks for a healthy and nutritious body. Let's take a detailed look at the five food groups as categorized by the USDA.

Fruits

The USDA recommends you consume a generous quantity of fruits every day. Now, you may choose to eat the fruit fresh, canned, pureed, juiced, or dried. All of these forms meet the USDA's fruit intake guidelines, but it is always best to consume fruits fresh. Canned and packaged fruits and juices often contain added sugars or preservatives. Fresh and raw fruits are always a better choice than processed fruits. Our bodies were built to digest and extract needed nutrients from food in its natural form. So, while the USDA can offer some informative guidelines, remember that not all fruit products should be treated equally.

Fruits are known to be low in fat and sodium, amounting to fewer calories for every serving. Although, fruits are inherently sweet to taste, they contain natural sugars and are quite beneficial for good health. In addition to this, they contain zero cholesterols, making it an obvious choice of indulgence for that sweet tooth. Remember the essential nutrients we spoke about a while before? Well, it turns out that fruits are rich sources of several essential nutrients such as potassium, dietary fiber, vitamin C and the all-important folic acid. Fruits such as banana, prunes, oranges and peaches are rich in potassium, making them important for maintaining healthy blood pressure levels. Fruits are also rich in dietary fiber and are known to reduce the risks of heart disease. In addition to this, fiber aids digestion, leading to better bowel functions. What's more, a small bowl of fruits can leave you feeling satiated and full at the same time. Fruits are rich in Vitamin C which is known to aid the growth and repair of cells and tissues. It also helps heal wounds and keep your teeth and gums looking healthy and gleaming. We must obtain Vitamin C from the food we eat because the human body is unable to synthesize it. It is a crucial vitamin for so many of the body's functions.

The amount of fruit recommended by the USDA varies across different age groups and genders. On average, children up until the age of 13 are should consume 1-1 ½ cups of fruits per day while adults from the age of 14 up until 60 should consume up to 2 cups a day. These should be thought of as general recommendations because everyone is a little different, and there is no one-size-fits-all plan. While the consumption of fruits comes with loads of benefits, many demonize fruits because of their sugar contents. If fruits are your only source of sugars, more than the USDA recommended amount will not hurt. However, it is important to note that individuals suffering from diabetes or an ailment that requires specific dietary monitoring should consult their doctors before consuming the recommended levels listed above.

Fresh fruit or fresh fruit juices contain a certain amount of water, but dried fruit pulp is devoid any water and amounts to a higher fruit quotient. For this reason, while adhering to the above levels of fruits, we suggest you equate every 1 cup of fresh fruit or fresh fruit juice to ½ a cup of dried fruit pulp. Similarly, fruits that have a noticeable amount of water in it can be consumed in larger quantities. So, the next time you intend to eat fruits such as watermelon and muskmelon, plate up a generous serving for yourself. The extra bit of serving will do you a world of nutritious good.

Vegetables

Any form of vegetable, whether consumed raw or cooked is considered to be extremely beneficial for good health. Vegetables can be frozen, dried or canned, but fresh, raw vegetables will deliver the most in terms of needed vitamins and minerals. One of the biggest steps any person can take to improving their health is to find a way to work more vegetables into the diet. Ideally, vegetables should comprise the largest portion of most of your meals.

Vegetables, like fruits, are low in cholesterol and rich in fiber, meaning that they work hard at eliminating heart and blood pressure-related diseases while aiding healthy digestion and bowel functions. They are also rich in potassium which helps maintain healthy levels of blood pressure. Foods such as potatoes, white beans, and soybeans are rich in potassium and, when consumed in limited quantities, aid a healthier body. While most vegetables can and should be consumed in large servings, it's better to limit white potatoes because they are so starchy. Try eating purple potatoes that have the same flavor, but pack a few more antioxidants than their white counterparts.

Many vegetables, such as carrots, have enough Vitamin A to keep your eyes healthy. What's more, they also prevent unforeseen infections and allergies. Whether consumed raw or cooked, vegetables amount to fewer calories than other foods and aid in achieving ideal weight management. Considering they are low in calories, they should act as your go-to foods to drive away any hunger pangs without the feeling of guilt. It's almost impossible to overeat when consuming vegetables. Plating a good share of vegetables of different colors ensures you are getting a wide range of healthy nutrients. In addition to its appealing appearance, each color signifies a specific nutrient group. For this reason, when you plate up a share of differently colored vegetables, you are ensuring you get a well-balanced variety of all the nutrients required for supreme health and wellbeing.

Tips for Selecting the Healthiest Vegetables

We've taken our advice a step further by giving you tips to choose vegetables of the highest nutritional value.

Only buy vegetables that are fresh and in season. This will ensure you buy them when they are at their best both in taste and nutrient content. What's more, the fact that they are in season makes them available in larger quantities so they cost comparatively less. You may choose to store frozen vegetables for quick and easy consumption. Frozen vegetables, when thawed in room-temperature water, are nearly as good as fresh vegetables. However, while there is no harm in eating frozen vegetables, we suggest you only do so when required. Using freshly bought vegetables takes the taste and nutritional value of the dish to the next level. And, keeping those veggies tasty is a big part of switching to a healthier lifestyle! If you are vegan, we suggest you select vegetables that are rich in potassium to make up for the lack of meat intake. Including vegetables such as sweet potatoes, beets, soybeans, lentils and kidney beans will give you the nutrition you need. While you can use canned vegetables, try and include more fresh vegetables in your diet. Canned vegetables are preserved in liquids that contain added salts. High levels of sodium consumption can increase blood pressure. Some vegetables, tomatoes in particular, will absorb harmful chemicals from cans or plastic containers. Eating fresh vegetables protects you from ingesting any harmful substances from packaging.

Grains

It's always easy to identify foods that fall under this group. As the name suggests, this type of food has a grainy texture to them. Foods made from wheat, oats, cornmeal, cereals and barley all fall under this category. Whether you wish to have them as breads, pasta, tortillas or cereals, grains are a great source of nutrition and should be a part of your diet.

Did you know that grains are categorized into two main subgroups? Depending on the type of processing and the grains they contain, they are divided into either whole grains or refined grains. While whole grains consist of the grain kernel, the bran, germ and the endosperm, refined grains are milled to separate them from the bran and germ. A good way to identify the two is to check out their texture. Whole grains are chunkier in appearance; some examples being oatmeal and brown rice. Refined grains, on the contrary, are smoother in texture and have a rather extended shelf life when compared to their counterparts. Some examples of refined grains are white flour, also known as all-purpose flour, and white rice. While refined grained might be more appealing to look and taste, they contain less fiber, iron and Vitamin B, making them harder to digest and lacking in their full nutritional potential. Although the process of refining grains requires them to be stripped of their fiber, iron and Vitamin B content, most of these grains are put through an additional process that replenishes the lost vitamins and nutrients, with the exception of fiber. It is always best to eat whole, unrefined grains. Getting vitamins and minerals that occur naturally in whole grains is much more beneficial than getting them from refined, enriched grains.

Similar to that of vegetables and fruits, the amount of grains to be consumed varies across different ages and genders. The USDA recommends that children aged 3-14 years should consume 3-5 ounces of grains while adults can consume anywhere between 6-8 ounces. It is common for most people consume more than the recommended quantities of refined grains through bread, pasta and all things that spell fast-food. However, we suggest you reduce your intake of refined grains and increase your intake of the whole grains. Ideally, all refined grains should be replaced with whole grains in the diet.

Grains are considered the warehouse of vitamins and minerals. They are rich in Vitamin B and consist of a high amount of thiamine, riboflavin, niacin and folate. They are also rich in iron, magnesium and selenium minerals, giving you a wide variety of vitamins and minerals with every bite you take. Whole grains are rich in dietary fiber, aiding digestion and bowel functions. In fact, this is one food that most nutritionists suggest while on a weight management program. Fiber acts as cleanse in your digestive tract. Maintaining a well-functioning digestive tract is important for maintaining a healthy weight and body. Consuming whole grains on a regular basis can help reduce your risks of heart disease and unsafe levels of cholesterol.

Protein

Proteins are essential for the development and growth of our body. They are composed of smaller compounds of amino acids, one type of essential nutrients we discussed earlier. While proteins are smaller, complexly formed compounds of amino acids, they do not complete the amino acids family altogether. We shall talk about amino acids and their role on our bodies in the next few chapters.

Proteins are the building blocks of our muscles and are responsible for a lot of our physical movements. Foods such as poultry, meat, soy, seafood, eggs, nuts and beans are all rich in protein. While children aged 2-13 should consume 2-5 ounces respectively; children aged 14-16 can consume up to 6 ½ ounces of protein. Adults too can consume anywhere between 5-6 ½ ounces of protein in a day. Different sources of protein have different effects on health and should not be treated equally. For example, red meat contains a lot of protein, but that does not mean it is an overall healthy choice. There is a common assumption that protein, no matter what form it comes in, is always good and more is better. This could not be further from the truth. Protein is an essential part of a healthy diet, but care must be taken when choosing how to obtain protein.

Foods such as beans, fish, eggs, and nuts are rich in protein and have the nutrients that help and maintain overall health. Foods high in protein are also rich in vitamin B and E, zinc, iron and magnesium. Protein in the diet aids protein synthesis, a process that helps build muscle while promoting tissue, cartilage, skin, and bone growth.

One drawback in consuming food rich in protein is that although they are highly beneficial for good health and overall body maintenance, some food sources rich in protein contain saturated fat and cholesterol that can result in health problems. For this reason, while consuming foods rich in protein, we suggest you keep track of the quantity consumed. Much less meat is required than what is typically served in the American diet in order to get needed amounts of protein. Foods that are rich in protein and saturated fat increase the levels of bad cholesterol in the blood. Bad cholesterol, also known as low-density lipoprotein (LDL), increases your risk for heart-related problems. Foods such as red meats are very high in saturated fat, immediately increasing your levels of LDL beyond the recommended healthy limits. Red meats include beef, lamb, hotdogs and bacon, to name a few. We suggest that you limit your intake of red meat and instead choose poultry meat or seafood as a healthier choice. However, if you are a hardcore non-vegetarian and love your red meats, we suggest you make the sensible choice of switching over to poultry or seafood. Seafood is rich in several nutrients. It consists of the all-important omega 3-fatty acids, known to promote superior health and vitality. What's more, they are very low in cholesterol and saturated fat and can be had without the worry and guilt of indulgence. Nuts are rich in protein content. Munching or snacking on nuts regularly can help prevent heart related problems in the long run. We also suggest that you choose raw, unsalted nuts instead of the fried, salted and artificially flavored ones.

Tips for Making Healthy Protein Choices

While choosing your source of protein food, choose foods that are low in saturated fat. If you are a non-vegetarian, we suggest you choose lean meat, poultry and seafood as your protein sources. Meats are inherently rich in fat, so it is advised that you avoid frying them. Avoid processed meats. Choose fresh meat instead. Processed meats, including deli meats, contain all kinds of additives that are of no benefit to your body. Snack on raw and unsalted nuts instead of fried and salted ones. Avoid anything processed as they are usually preserved in artificial liquids that when consumed over a long duration of time, can result in adverse effects on your health.

Dairy

Milk and all foods made from it fall into this category. Most dairy products are inherently rich in fat and calcium. While the calcium content present in dairy products is beneficial for bone and muscle growth, it is important to remember that dairy is high in fat. However, it is important to note that not all dairy products are rich in calcium and calcium can be obtained from other, healthier, vegetable sources. Foods such as cream cheese, plain cream and butter have little or no calcium content.

Despite the USDA's recommendations, it is not necessary to consume dairy to get any of the nutritional benefits associated with it. Calcium, fats, and proteins can all be obtained from healthier sources. A large portion of adults are lactose intolerant because consuming dairy beyond the early developmental years of childhood is not necessary.

Chapter 3- Serving Sizes

Now that you know the five food groups in detail, you should be well informed in making better food choices. A quick tip would be to vary the foods you eat. This will keep you interested while addressing key nutrients required for good health at the same time. Remember that you should combine a good mix of the food groups as no single food type will provide you with all the nutrients you require. Therefore, shuffle them a bit such that you soak in the goodness of all the nutrients and still manage to have the interest to continue your healthy habits.

Ok, so now for the obvious question: How much of the food we consume actually counts as the recommended serving? Well, call it the law of greed but more often than not, we end up indulging in a little more than the recommended levels of certain food types. We understand this tendency and have listed below the recommended serving size depending on the food types. So, while it is advised to consume certain foods within restricted levels, it's okay to indulge in some. The below list tells you what you can indulge in and what you cannot, making your choices a lot less complicated.

Restrict Breads, Pastas and Cereals

These foods are rich in carbohydrates, meaning that they have a high amount of calories and energy that can end up as fat deposits. Making sensible food choices, while adhering to the recommended levels of these foods will help you maintain overall good health. The recommended portions of the foods are:

- 1 slice of bread, preferably whole grain

- ½ cup of steel-cut oats
- 1/3 cup of cooked brown rice

Remember that if we you intend to load the above foods with cheese and meat, we suggest you plan ways to burn off the additional calories.

Indulge in Generous Servings of Vegetables

You simply cannot eat too many vegetables. They are your go-to food choices for a healthy and nutritious life. Vegetables are rich in fiber. Although fiber is a type of carbohydrate, it is one that you would want to include in your diet. Fiber aids digestion and works wonders at maintaining overall health and ideal body weight. So go ahead and serve up some greens and vegetables. The recommended minimum portions of vegetables are:

- 1 cup of raw leafy vegetables. You may also choose to cook them lightly if you want
- ½ cup of raw or cooked vegetables
- ¾ cup of vegetable juice

Now, although we mentioned the above quantities, it is perfectly fine to go a little beyond these recommended daily servings. Vegetables, whether eaten cooked or raw amount to fewer calories than other foods.

Fruits are Great Snacks

Well, by now you must already know the exceptional benefits of fruits to your overall health and body. So, go ahead, indulge your sweet tooth and appetite with a good share of fruits. The recommended daily portions of this food are at least:

- 1 cup of diced apple, banana or orange
- 1 cup of fresh fruit juice
- ½ cup of dried fruit pulp

Limit Your Intake of Dairy Products

Well, we understand just how tough this one might be. Think about it, most of the good things in life come from a glass of milk. Chocolates, yogurt, cheese, desserts are all dairy products. Although they indulge your taste buds like nothing else and have the power to drive away many woes, they also have the calories to worry you sick later. So stay wise and only have them within the recommended levels. The recommended portions of the food are:

- 1 cup of fresh yogurt
- 1 to ¼ ounces of natural cheese. Stay away from the artificially flavored ones

Protein Servings

Protein is important for building muscles in our body. We all require a certain amount of protein to carry on our daily activities. Poultry, fish, meat, nuts, and eggs are rich in protein and should be consumed within the recommended levels. The recommended limits of daily protein consumption are:

- 3 ounces of cooked meat, preferably lean meat, poultry or fish

- ½ cup of soya or dry beans
- 1 egg a day

Chapter 4- Understanding Proteins and Amino Acids

We've discussed the importance of the five food groups and the role they play in health and wellbeing. Now, let's take a look at one group a little more in detail: he protein group. Most of you might already know that protein is a complex combination of compounds obtained from different amino acids. You are probably wondering why they are considered so important and what good they do for your body. Well, we've tried to put things into perspective by answering all your queries on proteins and amino acids in general. This chapter highlights the importance of protein in your diet while educating you on the best sources of protein available in your food.

So, that brings us back to your question: Why is protein considered important, and what good does it do to your health and body? Protein helps your immune system function efficiently. Your immune system is solely responsible for keeping you healthy and active; the stronger your immune system is, the lower your risk of health-related issues. In addition to this, protein protects your skin, hair and nails from bacterial attacks and decay while providing your body the nutrients it requires to produce necessary enzymes.

You are what you eat! Your external body and the way you feel inside emulate and reflect your overall health and wellbeing. Being in tune with your body and its responses will help you identify an oncoming health adversity sooner than it can affect you. Symptoms such as muscle loss, weight loss, tiredness, breathlessness, frequent illness, and slow or stunted growth are all signs that your body is not getting or absorbing the required levels of protein from food. Recognizing such symptoms and testing the levels in your body might help you overcome a deficiency or disease before it gains control over your body. What's more, adhering to required levels of proteins, amino acids, and other nutrients will help bounce off infections and diseases coming your way, keeping you healthier for longer.

In the earlier chapters, we told you about the essential and non-essential amino acids. Let us understand them a little more in detail now. The reason doctors and nutritionists emphasize the consumption of protein is because protein provides your body with the amino acids it requires to build and maintain muscle tissue. Typically, amino acids are categorized into two types: the essential and the non-essential amino acids.

Essential amino acids are those that your body cannot produce by itself. These must be obtained from the food you consume. Conventionally speaking, there are a total of eight amino acids essential for healthy living namely: isoleucine, leucine, methionine, lysine, threonine, phenylalanine, valine, and tryptophan. However, recent studies have revealed that a possible ninth amino acid could be included in this list. 'Histidine,' an amino acid that our body struggles to produce on its own, has proved to play a significant role in aiding good health. Hence, there is an on-going debate to consider it as one among the other eight essential amino acids.

Non-essential amino acids are those that your body produces plenty of, and some believe that there is no need to obtain them externally. Some of the non-essential amino acids are glutamate, taurine, serine, tyrosine, alanine, arginine, proline and aspartate. While we agree that these amino acids can be synthesized and produced by the body, we also recognize that this might not be the case all the time. For example, a person suffering from an ailment that prevents his body from producing the required levels of the so-called 'non-essential' amino acids might in fact have a depleted stock of the nutrients, suggesting that what might be considered as non-essential to others might become essential to this individual. Similarly, a person living amidst highly toxic conditions might end up having inadequate levels of glycine in his or her body. For this reason, we believe that it is safe to consider all amino acids as essential and important. Following a diet that has a balanced amount of all the amino acids required by your body will help you avoid any unforeseen health problems.

Remember that your body can produce protein only when it has the required quantities of essential and non-essential amino acids. If your body is deprived of even one type, your body will not be able to produce the recommended levels of proteins it needs. This condition can lead to a multitude of problems. If your body is unable to produce the required quantities of protein, it will end up breaking down protein from muscle fibers, resulting in unhealthy weight loss, fatigue, and other health problems. It is imperative that you take the necessary steps to plan out a diet that is rich in all the amino acids. Although it is practically impossible to sit and manually track the amino acids you consume, consuming a healthy of fresh foods will ensure you are well covered and are within the recommended levels.

The Function of Protein

Generally, carbohydrates and fats are the first nutrients used as sources of energy. Once the levels of the two nutrients are exhausted, the body generates additional energy from the protein present in it. In addition to this, the body breaks down protein compounds into tiny amino acids that are then used to produce more protein. This protein that is produced and synthesized by the body is used for multiple physiological functions such as:

- Synthesizing the production of several essential proteins. The body is capable of manufacturing essential proteins such as myosin, collagen, keratin, and actin. These proteins aid healthy, muscles, tissues, bones, nails and hair growth.

- Secretion of hormones and enzymes required to maintain ideal sugar and blood pressure levels in the body. Enzymes act as catalysts to several chemical reactions that take place in your body. Without them, your body will not be able to function and perform as efficiently as it does. What's more, protein produced by the body further synthesize hormones such as insulin, glucagon, and thyroid.

- Transporting essential nutrients to tissues and muscle fibers. Did you know that some of the protein the body makes is responsible for transporting essential nutrients and substances to various muscle fibers and tissues? It produces haemoglobin, a protein responsible for making red blood and transporting oxygen, transferrin which is a protein that transports iron, ceruloplasmin which is responsible for carrying copper and other retinol-binding proteins that transport Vitamin A. Well, this is just the tip of the iceberg when it comes to the various functionalities of body-made protein; there are several other proteins that are responsible for various functionalities occurring in our body.

- Producing the required quantities of antibodies responsible for fighting against antigens such as bacteria and virus. By attacking the antigens, antibodies make them weak and visible to the immune cells. Once detected by the immune system, the antigens are destroyed and dealt away with in quick time; leaving you healthy and strong for long.

- Maintaining the required levels of fluid in the body. Bodily made proteins are responsible for maintaining the osmotic pressure in the body. By doing so, they help control and maintain the water levels present in our cells.

- Combating acid refluxes. Proteins can combine and link with both acidic and basic substances. This helps dilute any imbalance in acid or base concentrate, thereby overcoming the condition of acid reflux by maintaining the right balance.

Cooking Protein

Let us look at the impacts of cooking, storing and processing foods that are rich in protein content.

Have you ever wondered about the reactions that take place behind cooking up your favorite dish? Let's take the classic omelet for example; did you know that proteins from eggs, when beaten and cooked, go through a physical transformation called denaturation and coagulation? Sure, to the naked eye, an omelette can only look different in color, shape and size; but in reality and behind the surface level of the dish is an incredible process of protein breakdown and rebuild. Proteins when cooked or disturbed in any way break down and go through a process of denaturation in which they change in shape, decreasing the solubility of the protein compound in the process. However, when they go through the process of coagulation, the protein compounds clump together to rebuild in form and structure. Overcooking or heating protein rich food can disturb and destroy heat sensitive amino acids, making it difficult for them to rebuild into proteins.

Factors that Contribute to Protein Deficiencies

Protein is relatively hard to digest and is collectively absorbed and digested by the stomach, pancreas, and liver. First, the stomach secretes hydrochloric acid that helps fragment protein for easy digestion. The pancreas then kicks into action and secretes enzymes that help in further breakdown of protein compounds. Finally, the liver regulates and controls the absorbents, controlling the metabolism of amino acids from protein.

Now, while all this might happen in an almost auto-pilot mode; certain medical conditions that hamper the functions of the stomach, pancreas or liver might negatively impact the above process. In addition to this, bodies that are unable to secrete the required non-essential amino acids also hamper the process of protein absorption and digestion.

Protein Interactions

Now that we now the physical transformations and the process of digesting protein, how about its interactions with other nutrients? Simply put, how do other nutrients interact with protein? Well, it turns out that the levels of protein in your body impact the functions of various other nutrients, too. We already know that protein acts as a nutrient carrying vessel, transporting vitamins and minerals to various muscle fibers and body tissues. So when there is an inadequate amount of protein present in the body, there is impairment in the transportation and functionalities of the other nutrients.

Protein-Related Health Conditions

Although protein is considered vital for healthy bodily functions, an overdose of protein intake may have negative implications. Patients suffering from intense physical trauma, burnout and exhaustion are often advised to consume a high dietary intake of protein. On the contrary, patients suffering from thyroid and other weight related problems tend to accumulate more than the required levels of protein, resulting in fat deposits. They are advised to monitor their dietary intake of protein such that it stays within the recommended levels.

Foods Rich in Protein

While planning your dietary intake of protein, it is important to know which foods contain protein and which do not. This will help you stay informed and equipped for making better choices. Let us look at a few food sources that are rich in protein content. Most meats including red meats, poultry and seafood are rich in protein. However, when comparing their fat content, we suggest you opt for healthier choices such as tuna, shrimp, fish, and poultry over red, fatty meats. Red meat when eaten lean and in strict moderation is apt for protein intake. In addition to this, mushrooms, eggs, broccoli, cauliflower are great for protein intake. Legumes such as lentils, kidney, pinto, and garbanzo beans too are rich in protein intake for the vegetarianism. Even if you are not a vegetarian, it is good to try and achieve a healthier protein intake through vegetables and legumes while keeping the consumption of meats relatively low.

While addressing food sources of protein, doctors recommend you choose complete proteins instead of the incomplete protein types. Complete proteins are foods that provide all the essential amino acids listed earlier while incomplete proteins are those that lack a few essential amino acids. Eggs, meat, fish and poultry all fall into the category of complete proteins and are easy sources of essential amino acids. However, whether or not you are a vegetarian, we suggest you include beans, grains, nuts, seeds and a wide array of fresh green vegetables in your diet.

Nitrogen Balance

Nutritionists say the recommendations of dietary intake of protein vary from person to person. However, in general it is calculated with regards to the concept of nitrogen balance. Protein contains nitrogen. While digesting and breaking down protein, a certain amount of nitrogen is expelled. It is said that by continuously consuming enough protein, you end up excreting the required levels of nitrogen, balancing the levels of nitrogen in your body. Most adults are advised to maintain an ideal balance of nitrogen inferring that the quantity of nitrogen consumed through protein rich food is subsequently expelled out of the body. However, children and pregnant women are advised to maintain a positive nitrogen balance as it aids body growth and development. A body is in positive nitrogen balance when the nitrogen levels consumed through diet are higher than the levels expelled. A certain amount of nitrogen remains in the body to promote body growth and development.

Chapter 5- Healthy Eating Guidelines

Because of the rising rate of obesity and chronic ailments due to inappropriate nutrition, it's time we review our eating habits and focus on a balanced and nutritious diet. In an attempt to help you make the right food choices, we've set forth a few healthy eating guidelines that when followed can help prevent chronic ailments and diseases.

The recommended levels of calorie and nutrient intake vary across different ages, body types, physical activities, and genders. For example, children are highly active and hence have different nutrition needs when compared to adults. Women undergo several body changes throughout their lives and have specific nutrition needs. On the contrary, overweight people might have lethargic and sedentary lives inferring they require fewer calories while active adults have greater caloric needs.

The Habit of Healthy Eating

Contrary to common belief, healthy eating is not about limiting your dietary indulgences and needs. It's not about staying unhealthily thin just so you can fit into the perfect image, nor is it about sacrificing and depriving yourself of the foods you love. Healthy eating is about identifying with your body and its needs; it's about making you feel and look great without the remorse of missing out on something special; it's about having the energy to enjoy the greater things in life; it's about staying happy and living a full and complete life.

The world of nutrition and food ethics can be quite confusing to some because every time you think you've come up with the perfect diet plan, you'll have someone telling you how inadequate or inappropriate it is for your goals. We choose to address this a little differently. So instead of judging what is right and wrong, we've come up with a few fool-proof tips that can clear out all the confusion that might surround your mind right now. While it might be easy to chalk out and come up with a diet plan that is flawless, we understand it's practically impossible to follow it down to its minute detail. The tips mentioned below lay out ground rules to follow. Sticking to the remits mentioned will help you maintain a well-balanced and nutritious diet while indulging on the occasional cheat day.

Healthy Eating Rule 1

Set realistic goals for success. While it might sound great to say you'll change into a healthier person overnight, the results might be intermittent and temporary. We suggest that you look at taking things one step at a time. Make lifestyle changes that work at creating healthier eating habits. Once you've worked out an environment that aids and encourages the change, you'll find it easier to fulfill your goals. Working towards a gradual change with dedication and commitment will help you make more permanent changes. Once you've done it long enough for it to become a habit, you'll find it takes little effort and focus to eat right and stay healthy.

Look at simplifying things. Monitoring your calories down to the very last morsel you consume can be time-consuming and painstakingly irritating, both to you and the ones around you. Instead, simplify things by incorporating a good mix of fresh ingredients that are recommended as nutritious. On days when you want to indulge, add in your favorite food and combine it with the recommended nutritious ingredients while reducing the total serving size of it. Doing so will help you address your indulges while sticking to the boundaries of nutrition and health eating habits.

The one thing that most people fail to do while eating is the thing that drives them to eat the dish in the first place. They fail to relish the food that's in front of them. Stay in tune with your feelings; focus on how you feel while eating. This will help you address any unnecessary guilt or remorseful pangs after indulging in a meal; leading to healthier food choices in the long run. The key here is to make small changes; every small change leads to another, amounting to a drastic change in your eating habits over a course of time.

No one is perfect. Make peace with your occasional indulgences. Remember that you don't have to perfect your act and completely let go of foods that you love. The key is to feel good, stay healthy and live long.

More often than not, we fail to recognize water as a food group in our diet. Understand that water constitutes to 70% of your total body mass. Water fills space in your stomach. Similarly drinking water when thirsty or developing a taste for water can actually make you feel satisfied and content, just like you would when you indulge in your favorite food. Your good habit of drinking enough water can help flush out toxins and leave you feeling hydrated and energetic. One common mistake that we often make is to mistake thirst for hunger. So, the next time you feel those ravenous hunger pangs, sip on some water instead, the time spent in drinking water will help you analyze if it was real hunger or mere thirst fooling you.

Good nutrition goes hand in hand with exercise and workouts. If you do not exercise enough, you will not be able to flush out toxins and burn excess calories. When you fail to exercise your body, you can still end up with diseases and ailments even though you might be eating right.

Healthy Eating Rule 2

Remember that it's not just what you eat but how you eat it that makes up for what you are. Eating and living healthy is not just a routine. In order to live and eat healthy you need to think healthy. For this reason healthy eating is more than overcoming the food cravings you have, and it's more than the food currently sitting on your plate; healthy eating is about how you feel about food. Do you look at food as something to give you company on your way back from office or as a source of nourishment that fuels your passion for life and its activities? Considering how you feel about food and altering your mindset to looking at food as a source of nutrition will help you make sensible food choices.

Make it a habit to eat with people and not alone in front of the TV or computer. When we socialize and engage with people, we share thoughts, notice each other's habits and are more often than not influenced by the people we surround ourselves with. Eating with loved ones or friends will help you stay conscious of your eating habits. On the contrary, when you choose to eat alone, in front of the TV or the computer, you are more likely to overeat and binge because it is easy to lose track of your eating.

The next thing to do is to chew your food several times, savoring its flavors and taste with every bite you take.

Most often than not, we tend to rush through our meals, gulping down large bites without savoring their tastes and flavors. When you do so, you are less likely to feel satisfied with the meal. For this reason, make sure you set work aside and spend a few minutes to savor your meals.

Listen to your body and learn to differentiate hunger from boredom. Yes, you heard us right, most often than not, we seek food as a solace or for the want of nothing better to do. Eating should not be your favorite pastime. Only eat when you are hungry, and your body needs the energy. A quick tip would be to sip slowly on a glass of warm water. Warm helps kill acidity while filling up space in your stomach. Do this often, and you'll be surprised to realize that what you thought as hunger all these days was, in fact, your thirst for water or fluids.

You've probably heard this several times by now, but plan your meals in such a way that you end up eating your heaviest meal at breakfast and your lightest during dinner. A healthy and sumptuous breakfast is the best way to kick-start an active metabolism. What's more, you have the entire day to burn down the calories. Doing so will help you boost your metabolism while retaining higher levels of energy throughout the day.

Have fruit for dinner. It's fine to go light and eat fruit for dinner. This may feel a little odd initially, but recognize that as your brain trying to trick you back into your unhealthy eating habits. Ignore the cravings with all the will power you can muster and opt for a bowl of fruit instead.

Healthy Eating Rule 3

Serve up a good share of colorful fruits and vegetables.

Ever wondered what it would be like to eat a rainbow? Well, follow this rule, and you'll have one to eat from your plate. We've already addressed the importance of fruits and vegetables in the food groups sections. They are nutrient dense, low in calories and are packed with the goodness of essential vitamins, minerals and nutrients. What's more, nutritionists say there is no harm in doubling the quantity of fruits and vegetables in order to fill up hunger space in your stomach, provided they are cooked with low salt and little to no oil. We recommend you lay out a rainbow of colors when it comes to choosing the right fruits and vegetables. A good way to identify their nutrient quotient is to look out for their color. Deeply colored fruits and vegetables that are darker in shade are rich in vitamins, minerals, and antioxidants. In addition to this, each color signifies a specific nutrient content. Although it might be impossible to remember them all, it is safe to say that by selecting a wide range of colorful fruits and vegetables, you are sure to have a balanced and nutritious diet. Here's a list of food we suggest you consume:

- Berries go extremely well with cereals and contain as low as 40-50 calories per serving. In addition to this, they are rich in fiber and antioxidants, and they boost your immune system.

- Greens are packed with potassium, zinc, vitamins, iron, magnesium and calcium. While most people stick to iceberg or romaine lettuce, we suggest you expand your options. Kale, mustard greens, broccoli, cabbage, and spinach are all excellent options to try out and keep salads from becoming boring.

- Sweet vegetables do much more for your health than their sweet flavor suggests. Vegetables such as corn, beets, carrots, yams, sweet potatoes, and onions are all inherently sweet vegetables. They naturally substitute for the sugar or sweetness in your food without adding to the extra calories. In addition to this, they are rich in Vitamin A, B5, B6, thiamine, niacin and many more nutrients that are beneficial to your body.

- Fruits, in general, are juicy, delicious and sweet to taste. They are rich in fiber and aid both in digestion and healthy bowel functions. What's more, fruits such as berries, oranges, and green apples are very high in antioxidants by nature and help fight cancer.

Healthy Eating Rule 4

Ensure you consume healthy carbohydrates and whole grains.

We've already discussed the benefits of carbohydrates in your diet. We've also told you the advantages of fiber in the diet. So, make sure you plate up a good share of healthy and safe carbs such as fiber and whole grains. They are rich in antioxidants and work at fighting against heart diseases, certain types of cancers and even help prevent the onset of diabetes. To make things easy for you, we've listed a few healthy and unhealthy carbs. So, stay informed and choose wisely.

Healthy carbs that are safe and good for your body include whole grains, green beans, fruits, and vegetables. These carbs are rich in fiber and help you digest food more easily. What's more, they keep you feeling full for longer while maintaining the ideal insulin and sugar levels in your body.

Unhealthy carbs that are bad and should be avoided are foods that are mostly refined. This list includes white flour, refined sugar, and white rice. We've already told about the process of stripping them of all their nutrients and fiber, making them difficult to digest. These unhealthy carbs are also the ones responsible for the increasing levels of insulin and sugar in your blood. So, although they might be tasty, recognize the detrimental implications they cause and stay as far away from them as you possibly can.

Consume a wide range of whole grains in your diet. Whole grains are easy to identify as they are darker in color and coarser in texture than their refined counterparts. Whole grains include brown rice, barley, wheat flour, millet, oatmeal, unrefined corn meal and quinoa. What's more, they make for a number of delicious recipes and feel great in texture, giving your dish an overall visual and palatable appeal. While looking for whole grain foods, search for the label that reads 100% whole grain as opposed to words such as multi-grain or stone ground.

Healthy Eating Rule 5

Stick to healthy fats while avoiding unhealthy fats. Remember the information about healthy and unhealthy fats we told you earlier in this guide? Well, memorize them in your head so that you don't end up with the wrong type of fat on your plate. Consuming healthy fats act as nourishment for the brain, heart, skin, hair and nail cells. In addition to this, most healthy fats contain omega-3 fatty acids called known to work extensively at reducing your risks to cardiovascular and memory related diseases.

A healthy diet that contains healthy fats can include monounsaturated fats such as fats from plant and seed oil. Olive oil is a good example of this type of fat. You can also consume avocados, nuts, and seeds in your diet.

Avocados are great in antioxidants and are considered to be a powerhouse of nutrients. They are rich in vitamins and minerals and aid healthy and glowing skin. As for their nutrition quotient, they amount to 160 calories for every 100 grams. Nuts are also considered to be a powerhouse of nutrients. Nuts such as almonds, peanuts, walnuts, cashew nuts, and hazelnuts aid healthy living. Almonds are rich in calcium and vitamin E content. Cashew nuts are rich in iron, zinc and magnesium content. Hazelnuts are rich in homocysteine, an amino acid that fights against heart related problems and Parkinson's disease. Walnuts are rich in antioxidants, help fight against cancer and are a great source of omega three fatty acids. In addition to this, they help to lower the bad cholesterol also known as LDL in your body.

Polyunsaturated fats are fats such as fats from seafood. Seafood such as salmon, mackerel, cod and sardine fishes are rich in omega-3 and omega-6 fatty acids. Vegetarians can opt for unrefined sunflower, corn, soybeans and flaxseeds.

Now for the unhealthy fats. Make sure you reduce and avoid unhealthy fats such as:

Saturated fat present in animal fat such as red meat. Foods made from full fat and whole milk.

Foods that contain trans-fat or any type of oil listed as "hydrogenated" such as vegetable shortening, cookies, candies, chocolates, deserts, fried food, baked bakery products fall into the category of unhealthy fats. As unfortunate as it might sound, most of the fast-food and tasty food that you eat is unhealthy in nature. So do yourself a favor and reduce your indulgences. Trans fats or hydrogenated oils lead to an almost instant spike in blood pressure.

Healthy Eating Rule 6

Reduce your sugar intake.

Ask anyone what their go-to food at times of boredom and lethargy is, and they'll often choose a form of carbonated sugary drink, candy or anything that has some amount of sugar in it. Although sugar might momentarily increase your energy levels and make you feel good about life and yourself, understand that consuming excessive sugar in the form of sodas, candies, sweets and cookies can result in the onset of diabetes, cholesterol and high blood pressure, which is something you'd much rather avoid we bet! In an attempt to help you make the right choices and say no to the wrong ones, we've listed some handy tips to follow.

Stay away from carbonated and sugary drinks. Sodas, fruit punches, and mocktails are all things you should stay far away from. It has been measured that as little as 12 oz of soda has as much as 12 teaspoons of sugar in it, which is way more than the recommended levels and enough to hit the panic button straight away! Try sipping on a glass of fresh lime water instead, it's tasty, and refreshing, doing your body a world of good in return.

Instead of buying sweetened yogurt, buy plain yogurt and add a little bit of fruit pulp to bring in some sweetness to the dish. You'll be saving yourself a few extra calories in return.

We understand that sweet craving can be difficult to resist. However, by making the right choices, you can indulge your sweet tooth while limiting the calories, too. So the next time you have the urge to bite into something sweet, try having fruit instead. Fruits are rich in natural sugars and will help satisfy the sweet flavor you are craving.

Recognize the synonyms for sugar. Sugar can be conveniently disguised using several other names. Remember that whatever form or name it takes, sugar is best avoided whenever possible. Some names that synonymously spell sugar are:

- Cane sugar
- Corn syrup
- Golden syrup
- Honey
- Brown sugar
- Jaggery
- Sucrose
- Fructose
- Glucose

Healthy Eating Rule 7

While discussing nutrition, we'd like to emphasize that it's important you obtain nutrients from healthy, fresh foods as opposed to obtaining them from a bottle of pills or supplements. There is nothing better than eating a meal made out of fresh fruits and lightly cooked or raw vegetables. Although it might take a bit of an effort from your side initially, we are sure that once you see the results in front of you, you will agree that the efforts were worthy in every sense. Vitamin supplements are fractionated, meaning your body cannot readily use the isolated supplement. Many vitamins must be coupled with other vitamins or minerals to be properly absorbed and utilized. Whole foods contain these perfect combinations naturally. Additionally, vitamin overdoses pose a real threat to health. Vitamins should be obtained from the food you eat.

Chapter 6- Summary

Finally, with all the information listed in this book, we are sure you are more than informed to make wise food choices. Remember that it is never too late to change! Take small steps towards developing healthier eating habits, and you'll soon realize the big difference it does to your health and attitude towards food. Think about the positive changes you are willing to make and go about implementing them right away. Slowly when you think you are ready to take your small changes a step further; step up and welcome the healthier ways with open arms and a positive attitude. However, do remember that changing unhealthy food habits that you've cultivated over the years will take some time and effort from you. Accept your failures as stepping stones. Learn from your mistakes and use the lessons learned to overcome the next hurdle. Lastly, remember that YOU stand to GAIN greater HEALTH and LIFE from the CHOICES you make.

Here's wishing you healthy and nutritious days ahead! Stay healthy and live long!

Printed in Great Britain
by Amazon